I0420182

Depression:

10 everyday techniques to overcome depression and live the life that you want

By

Shawn Rogers

© Copyright 2015 By Infinite Possibilities Publications

© Copyright 2015 By Infinite Possibilities Publications- All rights reserved.

This document is geared towards providing exact and reliable information in regards to the topic and issue covered. The publication is sold with the idea that the publisher is not required to render accounting, officially permitted, or otherwise, qualified services. If advice is necessary, legal or professional, a practiced individual in the profession should be ordered.

- From a Declaration of Principles which was accepted and approved equally by a Committee of the American Bar Association and a Committee of Publishers and Associations.

In no way is it legal to reproduce, duplicate, or transmit any part of this document in either electronic means or in printed format. Recording of this publication is strictly prohibited and any storage of this document is not allowed unless with written permission from the publisher. All rights reserved.

The information provided herein is stated to be truthful and consistent, in that any liability, in terms of inattention or otherwise, by any usage or abuse of any policies, processes, or directions contained within is the solitary and utter responsibility of the recipient reader. Under no circumstances will any legal responsibility or blame be held against the publisher for any reparation, damages, or monetary loss due to the information herein, either directly or indirectly.

Respective authors own all copyrights not held by the publisher.

The information herein is offered for informational purposes solely, and is universal as so. The presentation of the information is without contract or any type of guarantee assurance.

The trademarks that are used are without any consent, and the publication of the trademark is without permission or backing by the trademark owner. All trademarks and brands within this book are for clarifying purposes only and are the owned by the owners themselves, not affiliated with this document.

Table of Contents

Chapter 1
Introduction

"Depression is like a prison where you are both the prisoner and cruel jailer" Dorothy Rowe

Depression is a state of mind which is very commonly found. Though depression is just a mental state, it impacts much more than just the mental health of the person. Depression symptoms consist of reduced levels of concentration, increased fatigue which further leads to fall in productivity levels of person, this again links up with the high levels of guilt etc. Usually the symptoms of depression are all interlinked. This way, the problem itself makes the solution easier. If you start attacking one of the symptoms, along with right medication, then depression can easily be controlled.

Depression- Not just about mental health:

Today with all the increased stress levels, depression is turning into a problem that is beyond one's personal space. There are suicides which have been recorded as done because of depression, there are impulsive decisions taken by people to harm others because of high levels of depression. When we look into the statistics according to various studies carried on by the WHO, the numbers indicate an immediate need to action.

- ➢ There are more than 350 million people who are suffering from depression, worldwide.
- ➢ In another study conducted over 17 countries across the globe, it is concluded that 1 in every 20 persons, is suffering from depression or depressive episode.
- ➢ More than 1 million people commit suicide every year, due to depression. This number further translates to more than 3 thousand people committing suicide every day, globally.
- ➢ Even the young children are not an exception. Teenagers, who are affected by depression, tend to show extreme levels of anger and frustration which again is harm to themselves and the society around.
- ➢ Though most effective medication is already in place, there are very few percentage of people who avail this medication, before it is too late. While in few countries more than 50% of depression victims get medicines, in many countries it is only 30% and in few more countries it is not even 10%.

So why we are still facing this problem directly or indirectly, though we have the most efficacious medical system, and advanced counseling techniques are available? In most of the instances, people do not understand how to identify depression. Once identified, they will not be willing to call it out for treatment because of the social awkwardness associated with depression. This eBook will help you with guidance on how to identify depression in various age groups.

This book will also call out what are few effective techniques to help in healing the depression.

Chapter 2
Types of depression

It is extremely significant to understand the types of depression, in order to identify if a person is suffering from depression or no. Since the depression is not something that equals "one size fits all" condition, the treatment too will be different and highly dependent on the type of the depression. There are various types of depression, which will have various levels of impact on the one who is suffering with it. Here are different faces of depression.

Depression - multiple faces.

➢ Vascular depression: This is a very newly recognized variant in depressions. While it is a fact that depression contributes a lot to increased stress levels, vascular depression is one variant that closely causes cardiovascular issues. This type of depression is very often found in people who are aged 60 and above.

➢ Anxiety depression: This is a well known critical type of depression. High anxiety levels, sensitivity to certain things without apparent reason are the key symptoms in this type of depression. This sensitivity without reasoning often creates problem for the patient in accepting medication or counseling without any hesitation. A study reveals that more than 40% of depression patients suffer with anxious depression. Often it happens that anxiety disorder is mistaken with depression. However, there are few symptoms which differentiate both these disorders. With this given anxiety towards the medicines, patients tend to resist the medication for a longer period. To mitigate the damage, it is common practice to use tranquilizers along with the medicines.

➢ Atypical depression: Atypical depression is something that is impacting more than 10 million Americans today. In this type of depression, people usually are reactive. Psychiatrists who were dealing with these people found it easy to remind the patients about the positive incidents from their past and cheer them up. Though they were not successful all the time, they could achieve this in more than 50% of their attempts. Advanced level in atypical depression has severe symptoms like high levels of sensitivity to rejections, problems in work area, series of disturbed relations etc.

➢ Melancholic depression: Another form of severe depression, which eventually leads to hospitalization of the patient. People usually show lack of interest in doing any activity for themselves. In addition, they are too slow or too agitated. Usually these symptoms are aggressive during the morning hours and patient will slowly shows reduced appetite and loss of weight as well. To slow down risk further to just weight loss, usually these patients are admitted to hospitals and closely supervised.

When we talk about the duration that depression impacts the patients, we have two types again. One is the major depressive episode, which has all the depression symptoms but will not last for a longer time than two weeks time. Usually this occurs when the person is impacted by loss of people whom they love, breaks ups etc. Suicidal tendency is less in this type of depression as the patient doesn't remain in the same state for a longer time. 17% of people who are in this depression status attempt suicides. The other variant is called Persistent depressive disorder (PDD), with all the same symptoms but for extended period. People in this state, always tend to see the empty side of the glass, regardless how small portion is left empty. People are tending to show incorrect social behavior, excessive sexual desire, poor judgment etc during the stage of PDD.

So, when the symptoms are threatening and sometimes harmful, don't we have any weapon to fight against depression other than just getting hospitalized? Not really. Most of the depression cases can be handled and coped up well, with some simple self-help techniques. These tips are easy to follow and good to share. We will read those tips in coming chapters, in detailed.

Chapter 3
Depression – Causes

"Depression is not just being alone and sad. It's feeling nothing. It's not wanting to be alive anymore".

J.K Rowling

In many instances people do not realize they are being the victims of deadly depression. By the time they realize there is something wrong, their mind will start racing with the question as to why is it happening? Below are few of the evident things which eventually cause depression... So, if any of your friends are loved ones seem to be in trouble and if you find any of the below relevant points then, you know how you can save them!

- SAD (Seasonal Affective Disorder)

We all have deep connectivity with the climate around. However, few are strong enough to handle the climatic changes effectively and move on with the routine. But few are extremely sensitive to the climate changes and it directly affects their moods. Research says, more than 5% people in America, are suffering with SAD (Seasonal Affective Disorder), and among these 1% people are highly sensitive to summer season.

- Smoking

The linking in between smoking and depression is like the historical "egg or chicken" riddle. Many people say that they smoke a lot when they are depressed. But medical science proved that nicotine has few elements which disturb the neurotransmitter activity that happens in the internal brain tissues. Hence, if you see a chain-smoker with depression, now you know before rushing him to hospital probably you must work on the re-habilitation.

- Thyroid

When the thyroid gland could not create enough thyroid hormone in the body, it is called hypothyroidism.   One of the main responsibilities of thyroid hormone is to regulate the neurotransmitter activity. Hence, if it is lacking, it will further lead to depression. So as a first check when you have depression symptoms is to check if you have thyroid symptoms as well. Typical thyroid symptoms include constipation, cold sensitivity etc.

- Sleep habits

When you don't have enough sleep, our brain cannot replenish brain cells, and that could be one of the strong reasons for depression.

- Addictions

One of the key addictions in today's time that has strong influence on brain functioning is "Face book". Being continuously on chat rooms and various social networking websites is like spending time in a fairy tale which is in contrast with the real world. People who spend a lot of time on social networking websites are said to have many issues with real time partners and relations. In 2010, out of all the registered depression patients, more than 1.2% of people aging 16 to 51 are assessed to be addicted to face book. They spend inordinate number of hours on face book and are suffering with moderate to severe stages of depression.

- Birth Control Pills

In some women who have undergone severe levels of depression, clinical research found that they have high levels of progesterone which is caused by the oral contraceptives. It doesn't happen with all the women who use these pills. But yes, certainly with women who have the previous history of depression, there are chances of repetition. Hence, in these cases alternative contraceptives like diaphragm are suggested.

- Genetic reasons:

In few situations though everything is right, people are found to be suffering from depression. In these cases, with little research it is often found that the depression is genetic and existed in family history.

- Environmental reasons

In addition to all the above reasons, surroundings of the patient are the key drivers for depression as well. Sometimes severe levels of mental/physical abuse in childhood can cause depression and suicidal tendencies. In few cases it could be social reasons such as stress due to education, failure at work etc.

Chapter 4
How to identify depression in various age groups

One of the significant phases of treating depression is right identification. Many of the suicidal attempts in depression cases could have been stopped if they were identified in the right stage. The symptoms of depression vary from each age group to the other. Here are few important points.

Symptoms of depression in elderly people:

➢ *Being sad most of the time.*

➢ *Fatigue and unusual tiredness*

➢ *Lost interest in their regular tasks like reading or walking or listening to their favorite music.*

➢ *Isolation or wanting to be left alone.*

➢ *Weight loss/ loss of hunger*

➢ *Lack of sleep/ no sleep at all.*

➢ *Increased intake of alcohol or smoking*

➢ *Suicidal tendency*

When it is time for elders to be dependants, apparently depression attacks. In few cases it is also observed that a series of deaths due to age too creates depression in elders. There is another reason which is often observed that when the partner dies, the remaining elder loses the interest on life and tend to leave all those habits which they used to do with their partner. This slowly kills their appetite and interest on life.

Symptoms of depression in teens:

> - *Being sad and losing hope over their ambitions/ short time goals.*
> - *Irritated most of the times, sometimes for no reason.*
> - *cries very very often*
> - *facing issues in mingling with friends and people around*
> - *lack of interest in hobbies*
> - *sudden changing in food habits/ lack of hunger*
> - *agitation or high levels of aggressiveness*
> - *lowered self esteem*
> - *reduced enthusiasm*
> - *low energy levels*
> - *lack of focus*
> - *suicidal tendencies*

Teenage depression is found many times unattended promptly as parents tend to mistake it as adolescence. Very often when the kids turn teens, they try and find their first friends in parents. During depression state of mind, they tend to crave parents support in terms of more number of talking hours. If this is attended, the risk of suicidal attempt can very well be mitigated. Of course, depression will still need to be medicated and supervised by a medical expert.

Another reason why most of the teenage girls suffer depression is due to biological changes. When a girl or boy is not able to understand the physical changes that she is going through, it is observed that they get depressed.

A very common reason that is observed in today's teens that is pushing them towards depression is the stress. It could be the high expectations which are set by parents for the child's education, grading system in the educational institutions etc. There are instances where kids in teenage are incorrectly routed towards drugs, alcohol and smoking. These addictions will be followed by failure of resistance, and guilt further leading to suicidal tendency.

Symptoms of depression in Men and Women:

> - *playing blame game often*
> - *ego is inflated most of the times*
> - *Suspicious and guarded over petty things.*
> - *Create conflicts*
> - *Feel restless*
> - *Try to take the charge of everything around.*
> - *Difficulty in admitting when in doubt.*

> *Use alcohol, sports, sex and TV to self-medicate*

Though the symptoms of depression are same in men and women, there are few evident differences as well. For instance, seasonal affective disorder seems to be impacting women more than men. While men suffer from lack of sleep and lack of appetite, women suffer with excessive sleep and over eating followed by weight gain and guilt. In few cases it is proven just opposite as well. In women depression is often closely associated with menopause, hormonal imbalance and aging as well. Women often found in depression post maternity due to the fact that the attention they were given till then, is suddenly routed to the new born. This sometimes gets serious but very often it can be cured without medication, with proper emotional and moral support from family.

 While it is difficult to deal with depression in women, with men it is difficult even to identify. Men usually do not open up and that makes it very difficult to understand what they are going through. Sometimes a simple stress at work could have been mistaken as depression as men do not easily come out and tell the people around as to what is happening with them. In few of the cases when men reach 40's, they tend to get into a state of mind where they think it's all over and they have done nothing in their life. This is when the depression symptoms are tend to show up more aggressively pushing them towards any nasty mistake. Sometimes it could be a sexual aggressiveness or sometimes it is a suicidal attempt as well.

Bipolar Disorder

Bipolar disorder is one of the mental disorders which are often mistaken as depression. BPD (Bipolar Disorder) is not depression, but certainly it can further lead to manic depression. BPD is nothing but high frequency mood swings. People who are happy right now may turn sad or angry in next minute. It could be vice-versa as well. What triggers this sudden mood change? It could be a random memory from past, or an unknown fear that is coming from future plans.

Why is it serious?

Ignorance makes it serious. Usually people fail to read the symptoms and warning signs of BPD, and hence it turns into serious levels of depression. During Bipolar, patients are observed to have two types of moods. One is manic episode and the other is depressive episode. During manic episodes, a person is usually highly charged up. They tend to spend a lot, even if they have to use their credit cards. During the depressive episode, they tend to be the opposite. They sleep excessively and still feel tired. In few instances, they won't be able to get out of their bed as well.

If these symptoms are ignored for a long time thinking it is just a physical tiredness, then chances are that the mental state may change into something even more serious.

Common symptoms in both the manias are as below.

- high levels of optimism or irritability
- unrealistic expectations around others
- High energy levels or too low energy levels.
- Quick conclusions.
- Lack of concentration
- Low judgment skills
- Recklessness about consequences
- Hallucinations and elusions

How to identify?

While it is extremely dis-heartening to see a loved one go through this phase, it is also important to be practical in gathering the facts before concluding that they are suffering with BPD.

- Keep a track on their moods.
- Check if their routine can be slightly changed, step by step. This way, you will know if the boredom is causing the mood swing.

- Check if there is any impact of SAD (seasonal affective disorder).
- Try and find out how things are going at their work place.
- Sometimes, it may also be possible that there is a problem with their education or friends, keep a check on that.
- Try and speak to a psychiatrist before you fix an appointment for them. An initial talk can always help in finding out the facts through an expert opinion.

When a person is under depression, it's not him/her alone suffering. It's the whole family, friends who suffer along with the person. No one would want to let go of a friend or family member just because of a mental state that has missed its order. While it is immensely important, to undergo medication to cure depression effectively, there are few things which a person need to adopt in order to help themselves.

In most of the cases, few simple techniques to set the daily routine can help fight the depression. As much as you fight instability and as much as you are stable, that effectively you can get rid of depression. It's just a long term mental status which is refusing to accept any positive thing about life. As a dying plant can be brought back alive just by care and nurturing, the same way a depressed mental state can very well be brought back to normalcy by few changes in lifestyle.

Depression has a lot to do with what a person does on daily basis. If their daily routine can be amended to increase positive outlook towards life, then it is a lot helpful in appreciating the things they already have in life.

When a person no longer is able to appreciate the supreme human life, they tend to get into suicidal tendency. When someone is not able to realize their self worth, they get depressed and tend to feel there is no point in living this life. So, as a friend or family, it is immensely important to make them feel what they are worth.

How to help a loved one fight depression:

"Self Worth comes from only one thing. Thinking that you are worthy" (Dr. Wayne Dyer)

- Change: Change their routine as much as you can. Help them start something new. A new thing can be as simple as gardening as well.
- Seek their help: Tell them they and only they can help you in a particular task. Let them work on it.
- Genuinely appreciate: once the task is complete, give them a detailed appreciation. A genuine feedback

would include why they were chosen to do that, how difficult the task would have become for others to complete and most importantly what is that one thing this person has in them to complete the task with ease.

- Motivate: If the task is incomplete, don't hurry and assign something else. Try to have a chat as to what is stopping them. Try to help them do it, instead of leaving it. Remember, if the person is leaving the task incomplete, it will increase their sense of negativity about self. Their sense of self worth will never come back at all.

- Drag them into your workout: It is important to have a physical work out for any person. Drag them for a walk, for a cycling session, for a work out session, for a running marathon or a simple jog. This way, you might also find an opportunity to talk them openly about what they are suffering with!

- Talk positive: talk to them about all positive things on the earth. Positivity is that one thing that can bring sunshine on any cloudy and gloomy day of life.

But what if the person wants to fight depression all by themselves? We will now read on, what are the self-help techniques one can follow on daily basis just to keep their mind busy enough so that the depression stays out of mind. It is important that the effort starts from one's self, instead of a friend or a well wisher.

Chapter 5
Depression-10 everyday techniques to overcome depression and live the life that you want

"The best self help one can do is wanting to be happy than being a victim"

Sidney Sheldon

Is it difficult to live the life you want? The answer lies in another question. Is it difficult to want the life you have, while keep aspiring for more? In many of the instances, we do not realize what it is being a human. Human life is the most powerful life in the universe. Only a human has ability to think and create. But unfortunately, because we have the ability to think, we have an option to think negative as well. That is the reason why depression is taking a toll over many lives. It is the awareness that makes it easy to fight against depression. The more you know about what creates it, the easier it is to fight against it. As we read before that, climatic changes, addictions, work stress, negative thinking are few vital reasons which cause depression, now it becomes easy to jot-down a plan for self, to fight against these causes.

Here are 10 questions that you should ask yourself and seek a solution from there to fight against depression.

1. Are you too busy?

We all love to be busy... Don't we? But do we all know what the difference is between being busy and being stressed? If we take our favorite coffee as an example, being busy is a full cup, being stressed is an overflowing cup. An overflowing cup can ruin the whole purpose of coffee. It ruins the look of it, since it's overflowing you can't drink it and hence, it's of no use!

So it is important, to understand where to draw the line. Try to adopt a checklist before you say yes to anything.

➢ How is my current schedule?
➢ Do I have 6-7 hours time for sleep?
➢ Do I have time for my work-out/ walking routine?
➢ Do I have time for my kid's assignments or collage workshop?

If all these are yes, then you can look at accommodating more work. By doing this, you are allocating time for your priorities, not other's priorities.

2. Am I addicted drinker or a social drinker?

The big one! While it is ok to drink occasionally, it is important to ensure that it is not taking a toll on your moods. If you are an addicted drinker, then you must know that alcohol is actually nervous system depressant. The price of alcohol is much more than what you pay to buy it. Here are few hard facts.

- ➢ Your nerves are weakening with alcohol.
- ➢ Your performance is at stake.
- ➢ Your leaves are more so your job is at risk.
- ➢ You lose your social image.
- ➢ Your financials are broken.
- ➢ As a whole, your mental stability is at stake.

So, by avoiding alcohol one can improve their day to a greater extent. Try and reduce the intake first and then slowly stop drinking it.

3.   What kind of company you are in?

It is important to keep surrounded by positive people in life. In many instances, the negativity in others influences us silently. It creeps into us, without knowing it. How do you know if the other person is being hard on you and your mental state? Here...

- ➢ Does this person make you feel insecure about them?

➤ Does this person makes you always feel they are way too good to be with you?

➤ Do they complain a lot?

➤ Are they unhappy in life, continuously?

If all these answers are 'yes', then you know why you are depressed. Just be away from these people and be happy. Be with someone who is with themselves and who are happy with you.

4. Do you realize the good things in life?

Very often, we do not realize what we have in life. In fact, we do not realize the life itself is the biggest treasure. Simple things like being able to get up and work, being able to eat on own, being able to walk around without assistance, being able to earn respectfully and earning respect all these are only few beautiful things about being human. Appreciate these things in life, in order to appreciate the life that is given to us, generously. To do this effectively, when you are out in a public place, observe people. What they do, how they talk, how they behave with others, how they are dealing with the family members. In many instances, you may realize what you have been doing in wrong or you may get a ground breaking idea on how you can change your behavior in dealing with your family.

5. Do you have a plan for next 2 years?

These short term goals are like fueling stations for the life journey. As much as you refuel it, that smooth the journey is. What happens when you are in a new place, without a map or a guide in hand? You get into fear, and that fear causes stress. The same fear of being worthless creeps into you, when you do not set your short term goals and keep working on them. No matter what happens, your goals should be your priority.

6. How does your day look?

It is essential to have a workout routine set for a person to be active. When you do not work out on daily basis, you cannot be sure of your health, your weight, and how you look. This uncertainty too causes stress. When you workout endorphins are more in your body and this boosts the positivity in brain functioning. Here are few tips not to miss the workout routine

➤ Keep a checklist in a place where you can often see. This checklist must have how many times you walked or worked out in a week.

➤ Keep it going for few weeks. Then it keeps alarming you if you are going down week by week. Mark it with red, so that you won't miss it!

> Drag a friend whom you are comfortable with, to the workout.

7. Do you eat healthy?

Eating healthy plays a vital role in helping the antidepressants do their job. It is important to keep a check on what you are eating on daily basis, to avoid foods which will boost depressants.

> Increase the intake of foods that contain fatty acids.

> Increase the intake of folic acid, vitamin B etc

> Spinach and avocado can help way high in increasing folic acids.

> Reduce the intake of sugar.

> Eating sunflower seeds, beetroot, leafy vegetables etc to cope up with the moods.

8. Do you sleep enough?

An adult requires at least 6 hours of sleep at a stretch in a day. This way, the anti-depressants are kept active and re-charged. This kind of sleep routine also helps the medicines to be effective.

> Ensure the place where you sleep has no distractions such as T.V, comp etc.

➢ Disconnect Wi-Fi before you sleep, so that nothing can really take your attention.

➢ Ensure you go to bed on the same time every day.

➢ If you can't sleep after all these, try and change your workout schedule or walking to evening times. Sometimes it's easy to fall asleep, with a tired body.

➢ Wake up early, even if you slept late. This way, by next day night, you will be tired and fall asleep quickly.

9. Do you contribute additionally?

It is important to contribute little little to the home, to the society in order to feel good about one's self. It could be planting trees, feeding the hungry, cleaning the premises, feeding the orphan animals anything... That will make you smile.

10. Most importantly, do you laugh enough?

The most important anti-depressant that one can use is a heart-felt laugh. Watch a lot of funny stuff, share jokes with your friends and family, make it interesting when you are talking using jokes in between, make it a habit to read at least three jokes a day, and share it with as many people as you can. All these things will make you feel good. Others will feel good too. It is immensely pleasing when we make others feel happy. Not all can do, if you can, then you have something in you!!

This life is too short to be sad and become complicated. Be thankful for the life, be appreciative of others' efforts, be genuine about feedbacks, be straightforward while saying NO, be kind when someone is broken, be empathetic when someone fails. There is one rule that will give a lot of mental peace, if followed in everyday life.

"Everyone you meet is fighting a battle that you know nothing about. So, be kind. Always"

Chapter 6
Epilogue

Depression is like a demon with many faces. There are varieties like depressive episodes, persistent depression, anxious depression, BPD (Bipolar Disorder) and more variants. While it is possible that it might attack people because of their jeans, most of the times depression is caused by stress, addictions, rough relations, loneliness, hectic schedules etc. Unfortunately, all these are the reasons which could have been avoided. Fortunately, these are all the reasons which can still be worked upon. So, it is just a moral support and motivation that is needed for one to get out of depression. While there are medicines which can work as anti-depressants, there are many natural techniques which can be used to fight the depression in a very effective manner.

Depression has no exceptions when it is about age groups and gender. Starting from kids to elders, men and women all are prone to depression depending on the environmental and genetical causes. It is difficult to ascertain if one is undergoing depression or stress just because they are sad. There are many symptoms which need to be tracked and observed for certain time and only then it can be concluded. Once done, while the psychiatrists are helping with the medication part, the patient needs a lot of self help. He / she also needs a lot of help from the family and friends in terms of moral and emotional support for effective healing.

Yes, there are instances where depression can lead to a permanent hospitalization but there is a long way to it. Meanwhile, it can very well be identified with symptoms like withdrawal nature, irritability, sadness, reasonless reluctance to do things which the person usually like doing, suicidal talks etc. When you spot these symptoms in yourself or in a loved one, be quick in acting on it. That way, you can mitigate the risk to a greater extent.

Keep a healthy routine that will include your favorite things, favorite people who can influence in positive way, eat healthy and workout well.

"We cannot change what we are not aware of. But once we are aware, we cannot help but change".
    Sheryl Sandburg

www.ingramcontent.com/pod-product-compliance
Lightning Source LLC
Chambersburg PA
CBHW062029280526
45787CB00005B/2261